Homemade Body Scrubs

52 All Natural, Simple &
Easy To Make Body Scrubs
Face Masks
Lip Balms & Body Washes

Table of Contents

Introduction

Are you ready to get rid of dull, rough or troubled skin and bring out your natural beauty?

Do you have good skin already but want to maintain and improve it even more?

If so this book is for you because it contains the absolute best, most sumptuous, pampering, healing and moisturizing body scrubs, face masks, lip balms and body washes that you will find.

My name is Lorraine White and I am a wife, mother, sister, daughter, aunt and friend. I am like most moms who juggle work and home life. I have three children so I am always looking to save time and money in all areas of my life.

About five years ago I started to make these wonderful salt and sugar based scrubs and they have not only saved me lots of money, I have seen how you can treat debilitating skin conditions very easily with the right scrubs and moisturizers.

I have given my scrubs away as gifts and often get requests to make up special batches for friends and family members. Over the years I have often been asked how I make them. Rather than keep writing down recipes and telling everyone individually I decided to compile my recipes to show just how simple and how rewarding they are to make.

I now want to share this book with you. It is packed with recipes for different types of scrubs broken down into five categories. You will find a fantastic variety of:

- Scrubs that heal
- Scrubs that moisturize
- Scrubs that refresh and revitalize
- Scrubs suitable for night time

1

- Super luxurious and indulgent scrubs

I have also included lots of recipes for some of my other homemade natural beauty products. These are my:

- Homemade face mask recipes
- Homemade lip balm recipes
- Homemade body wash recipes

If this is the first time that you are learning about how to make your own homemade beauty products, you are in for such a treat. You can look forward to more beautiful and radiant skin and that's just for starters.

Lorraine xx

What Are Natural Body Scrubs?

Homemade natural body scrubs are simply body conditioners made up of three to four of the most wholesome ingredients. These scrubs help to exfoliate, moisturize and soften your skin and with prolonged use can totally transform the complexion, tone and overall feel of your skin.

If you have dry or damaged skin, they can help to relieve the irritation that you feel, particularly in hot or cold weather conditions. Natural body scrubs are an alternative to using ready made scrubs that you buy in the store that are often full of hidden and harmful ingredients.

My body scrubs are super easy to make and I always say to people who ask, making body scrubs is a bit like making a salad, you toss a bunch of ingredients in a bowl, throw some oil on them, give them a stir and that's it, you have your very own body scrub that will works wonders on your skin.

What's great about these scrubs is that you can create a spa like experience right in the comfort of your home and you will only pay pennies compared to what you would pay if you booked into one of those fancy spas.

There are all types of homemade body scrubs that you can make, you can make them to treat particular skin conditions or simply make them in order to completely immerse yourself in luxury ingredients that are served to do nothing else but pamper you.

These scrubs are far more beneficial to your skin than almost anything you can buy off a shelf because they are made from 100% natural ingredients, no preservatives, no additives, no harsh chemicals, zilch, nada, nothing.

I like to use things that I have in the kitchen already and often make new body scrubs right off the bat as soon as the idea enters my head. The best thing about making my own products is that I know exactly what is in them which is invaluable to me.

Now that I know about these wonderful homemade luxury scrubs I simply cannot go back to using the store bought products that I used to put on my skin. I can neither subject my family members to all the rubbish that they put in those products so we all use natural homemade products in our house.

Please refer to the next chapter to read about some of the hazardous and harmful chemicals that are secretly hidden in some of those store bought products. I haven't purchased a store bought soap, scrub, body wash or any bathroom beauty product for the last five years. Since I started to make my own homemade body scrubs I haven't looked back and I have managed to save myself a small fortune at the same time. By the time you finish this book, you will hopefully not be in a hurry to want to buy any more of them either.

Hazardous Ingredients I Found In Store Bought Body Scrubs!

Five years ago I was motivated to start experimenting with and making my own homemade beauty products after finding out about all the harsh chemicals and toxins that are hidden in them. I learned that these toxins seep into your system through your skin and can have devastating effects on your health.

Did you know for example that some manufactures use the following toxic and harmful chemicals in their products:

- Synthetic (un-natural) fragrances
- Methlyparaben
- Oxybenzone
- Stearalkonium Chloride
- Diethanolamine
- Propylene Glycol
- Artificial colors

There are absolutely tonnes and tonnes of other harmful and toxic chemicals that they use too. I have only listed the few that I can remember. Look them up and compare them with the ingredients on your own products (if you have any store bought products) and I think you will be surprised!

I can barely even pronounce any of the toxins and I wonder why? When I found out what was going on that was it for me, I decided to make my own products so I knew what I was putting ON my body and IN my system.

I cannot stress enough the importance of knowing what you are putting on your skin. Make it a priority to examine the products that you currently use and cut out the ones that have these harsh chemicals in them.

List of Common Ingredients I Use & Their Health Benefits

Before I move onto the individual recipes, I would like to mention a few things first. In my true experimental nature I don't like to be too rigid and like to create my natural products in an organic way with the ingredients I have available at the time. I am imagining you are the same and would therefore like to say that you can adapt any of the recipes to suit your individual taste and budget.

Body Scrub - How much does each recipe make?

Most of the recipes in this book will give you enough for two applications. Some of the scrubs are for one. This is because I sometimes only like to make a quick scrub for the moment and therefore don't require as much in the way of salt, sugar, oil etc. Where this is the case you will see that I only use 1/2 cup measurements.

If you want to make more or less body scrub or you want a more solid or runny consistency for your body scrub then just experiment, adding more salt, sugar or oil to your recipe until you get the consistency that you like. It really is super easy.

In this chapter I want to briefly discuss some of the basic ingredients that I use and the health benefits for each and also give you some alternative options if you don't have the same ingredients to hand.

Salt (Used as an exfoliator)

I use sea salt or dead sea salt in most of my salt body scrub recipes. You don't have to stick to the salt I use though if you don't have any of that salt at hand. You can substitute the salt I use with the salt of your choice. Other salts you can use include:

- Table Salt
- Kosher Salt (bigger salt granules)
- Epsom Salt

Sugar (Used as an exfoliator)

In my sweet homemade body scrub recipes nine times out of ten I use just natural organic brown sugar. Again, you are not restricted to using this (or even using organic products) and can try any type of sugar like:

- Turbinado (raw) sugar
- White sugar
- Regular brown store bought sugar

Oil

You need a carrier oil to help bind the ingredients together and make the scrub easier to handle and spread over your body. Different oils have different skin benefits and you don't need to stick to one oil either. You can mix two oils in one scrub. If I use an oil that you don't have, you can replace it with any of the following:

- Almond Oil - Dry skin fighter full of E, A & D vitamins. Good for moisturizing and fighting the appearance of wrinkles.
- Avocado Oil - Fantastic skin boosting oil that is great for treating eczema and dry skin conditions helping to accelerate healing.
- Coconut Oil - Perfect moisturizing oil and one of the best skin softeners
- Grapeseed Oil - Good for oily and acne skin problems with known anti-aging properties
- Jojoba Oil - Good for oily skin types as it helps regulate oil production. It is a great moisturizer too and really good for stretch marks

- Olive Oil - Fantastic oil with anti-inflammatory properties. soothing and packed with skin enhancers and protectors.
- Vitamin E Oil - Great moisturizing and healing oil, good for treating scars and dark spots

Essential Oils

I use a variety of essential oils in the recipes in this book. You can stick with mine or use your favorites, it's your body scrub and it is entirely up to you. Some of the common essential oils I use are:

- Lavender oil - Wonderful oil and one of the most common. Great for both dry and oily skin and great for creating calming scrubs. Also very good for treating acne, wrinkles and tightening the skin.
- Tea tree oil - Natural anti-bacterial and anti-fungal oil, perfect for troublesome skin, acne, dermatitis and a range of other skin conditions.
- Chamomile - Calming and soothing oil with so many benefits. It is anti-bacterial, anti-fungal, is used as an anti-depressant and is great for making night time scrubs
- Geranium - This is a great stress relieving oil, it helps to relieve tension in your muscles and revive you. It is said that Geranium helps to balance you spiritually.
- Rose - Known for the effective treatment in toning and lifting the skin and fighting feelings of anxiety, thus putting you in a more relaxed state. It is also good for acne and dry skin conditions
- Lemon - Perfect for cleansing and cleaning the toxins found in your skin. It has anti-inflammatory properties as well so it can be used in a variety of scrubs. It is also totally refreshing and you definitely feel lifted with this oil.
- Neroli - Another anxiety and stress busting oil, it is great for the night time with its calming effects due to its high levels of natural sedatives.
- Peppermint - For oily skin types, this oil is also great if you are feeling a bit heavy (not in weight but in how you feel!). Great for treating itchiness and muscle pains as well.

Other Ingredients I use

- Yogurt - I use it to help remove dead skin cells on my body, it moisturizes and brightens the skin.
- Oatmeal - Great skin cleanser and restorer. Good for itchy and dry skin as it helps to lock in moisture.
- Nuts - Good for tired and problematic skin. Helps to bring back natural glow.
- Honey – It has been used for thousands of years to nourish the skin, honey helps to open up and unclog the pores on your skin..
- Aloe Vera Gel - Very calming, healing gel, good for treating dry skin conditions
- Herbs - The power of natural herbs are well known. I use fresh herbs in some of my recipes because of the wonderful powers each one has.
- Fruit - Same thing, the healing benefits of fruit on the skin are well documented. I love using fresh strawberries, lime, orange, apple, banana, anything really, as long as it's fresh.

Adding color to your scrubs

Personally I don't like to add any color to my scrubs and prefer them in their natural form however, you can add color if you wish. Some people like to add food coloring to give their scrub a richer color. Experiment and see what you prefer, remember it's up to you.

Storage of your natural body scrubs

Don't forget that we are not using any nasty preservatives in these recipes so the scrubs won't last more than a couple of weeks in my opinion. This is when stored in the bathroom. Storing it in the fridge will prolong the life of the scrub but it will also make the scrub hard and it takes too much time to soften it and use it to bother. It's quicker for me to just make them as I need them.

When you have made your products, store them in air tight containers or glass bottles for best results.

Please see the relevant chapters for storage tips on the other homemade natural beauty products in this book.

My Favorite Body Scrubs Recipes

I have so many body scrubs that I like to use and I am always experimenting with fresh fruits and different essential oils to make new body scrubs. I make body scrubs at least once a month and package them nicely to give away as gifts to loved ones all the time. You could do the same.

Who can resist a beautifully scented body scrub? These gifts are always so well received. My body scrubs have now become highly coveted gifts amongst my family and friends because they say they just can't get anything like this in the shops.

They know they are unique and luxurious products. They make wonderful presents and what's great about it is that they are so easy to make that you can whip one up in an instant.

There are literally thousands of different body scrub combinations that you can make. This book has enough to keep you going for quite a long time. Get ready to give your body the best pampering it has ever had.

Skin Conditioning Body Scrub

I love these recipes for my skin conditioning scrubs and use them often for a range of different skin complaints for myself, family and friends. Take a look and see which one you need to use on your skin first.

Cellulite Fighting Body Scrub

Ingredients Needed:

- 1/2 cup brown sugar
- 1 cup coconut oil
- 1/2 cup ground coffee
- 1 drop Juniper essential oil
- 1 drop Fennel Seed essential oil

Directions:

1. Put all the ingredients in a bowl and mix together.
2. Apply the scrub to your damp skin just after you have taken a shower
3. Leave it to work its magic for 5 minutes
4. Shower yourself clean
5. Dry yourself down and enjoy how much better your skin looks and feels

Magnificent Milk & Honey Body Scrub

Ingredients Needed:

- 1 cup oatmeal
- 3 tablespoons honey
- 3 tablespoons whole milk
- 3 tablespoons olive oil

Directions:

1. Put all the ingredients in a bowl and mix together.
2. Apply the scrub to your damp skin just after you have taken a shower
3. Leave it to work its magic for 5 minutes
4. Shower yourself clean
5. Dry yourself and enjoy how luscious your skin feels

Luscious Mango Body Scrub

Ingredients Needed:

- 1 cup brown sugar
- 1/2 cup chopped mango (chopped fine)
- 4 tablespoons coconut oil
- 2 drops rosemary essential oil

Directions:

1. Put all the ingredients in a bowl and mix together.
2. Apply the scrub to your damp skin just after you have taken a shower
3. Allow the scrub to soak into your skin for 5 minutes
4. Shower yourself clean
5. Dry yourself, relax and enjoy how nice your skin feels

Cleansing Cornmeal Body Scrub

Ingredients Needed:

- 1/2 cup cornmeal
- 5 tablespoons coconut oil (melt for 3-5 seconds in microwave if it is solid)
- 3 tablespoons whole milk

Directions:

1. Put all the ingredients in a bowl and mix together.
2. Apply the scrub to your damp skin just after you have taken a shower
3. Allow the scrub to soak into your skin for 5 minutes
4. Shower yourself clean
5. Dry yourself off and check out your luxurious feeling skin

Moisturizing Avocado Body Scrub

Ingredients Needed:

- 1 ripe avocado
- 1/2 carrot (grated as finely as possible)
- 2 tablespoons coconut oil
- 1 tablespoon sea salt

Directions:

1. Peel and mash the avocado flesh into a bowl
2. Add the carrot and sea salt and mix together
3. Add the coconut oil and mix into a spreadable paste
4. Apply the scrub to your damp skin just after you have taken a shower
5. Allow the scrub to soak into your skin for 5 minutes
6. Shower yourself clean
7. Dry yourself off and appreciate your beautiful skin

Restoring Raspberry Body Scrub

Ingredients Needed:

- 1 1/2 cups brown sugar
- 4 tablespoons coconut oil
- 4 tablespoons lavender essential oil
- 3 tablespoon grapefruit essential oil

Directions:

1. Put all the ingredients in a bowl and mix together
2. Apply the scrub to your damp skin in the shower
3. Allow the scrub to soak into your skin for 5 minutes
4. Shower yourself clean
5. Dry yourself, relax and enjoy how nice your skin feels

Super Quick Raw Body Scrub

Ingredients Needed:

- 1/2 cup sea salt
- 1/4 cup olive oil

Directions:

1. Put the salt and olive oil in a bowl and mix together
2. Apply the scrub to your damp skin in the shower
3. Allow the scrub to soak into your skin for 5 minutes
4. Shower yourself clean
5. Pat yourself dry and enjoy your naturally clean and softer skin

Healing Body Scrubs

Recipes that heal the skin are wonderful because you begin to feel the benefits of these ingredients almost as soon as they hit your body. Turn the page and get ready to heal that skin.

Therapeutic Neroli, Jasmin & Tea Tree Body Scrub

Ingredients Needed:

- 1 cup natural sea salt
- 1/4 cup Argan oil
- 1/4 cup Flaxseed oil
- 3 drops Jasmin essential oil
- 3 drops Neroli essential oil
- 1 tablespoon fresh crushed ginger

Directions:

1. Put all the ingredients in a bowl and mix together into a spreadable paste.
2. Apply the scrub to your damp skin just after you have taken a shower
3. Leave it to work its magic for 5-7 minutes
4. Shower yourself clean
5. Dry yourself and enjoy your beautiful skin

Tea Tree & Cucumber Cooling Scrub

Ingredients Needed:

- 3 cups sugar
- 1/4 cup olive oil
- 1/4 cup cucumber (shredded)
- 1 organic green tea teabag
- 1 drop Tea Tree essential oil

Directions:

1. Snip the green tea teabag and remove the tea from the inside, put it in a bowl
2. Add all the other ingredients to the bowl and mix together.
3. Apply the scrub to your damp skin just after you have taken a shower
4. Leave it to work its magic for 5 minutes
5. Shower yourself clean
6. Dry yourself off and enjoy

Raw Oatmeal Body Scrub

Ingredients Needed:

- 1 1/2 cups natural raw oatmeal
- 5-10 tablespoons warm water

Directions:

1. Put the oatmeal in a bowl and pour the warm water over it
2. Leave it to stand for 5 minutes until the oats have softened
3. Apply the scrub to your body and massage into your skin concentrating on the hard and rough patches like your knees and elbows
4. Leave it on your body for 5-10 minutes
5. Shower yourself clean
6. Dry yourself off

Soothing Aloe Body Scrub

Ingredients Needed:

- 3/4 cup sea salt
- 1/4 cup brown sugar
- 3 tablespoons coconut oil
- 4 tablespoons Aloe Vera gel

Directions:

1. Put all the ingredients in a bowl and mix together.
2. Apply the scrub to your damp skin just after you have taken a shower
3. Allow the scrub to soak into your skin for 5 minutes
4. Shower yourself clean
5. Dry yourself, relax and enjoy how nice your skin feels

Coffee Anti-Oxidant Body Scrub

Ingredients Needed:

- 1 cup Jojoba oil
- 1/2 cup ground coffee
- 1/2 cup brown sugar

Directions:

1. Put all the ingredients in a bowl and mix together.
2. Apply the scrub to your damp skin just after you have taken a shower
3. Allow the scrub to soak into your skin for 5 minutes
4. Shower yourself clean
5. Dry yourself, relax and enjoy how nice your skin feels

Dry Skin Smoothing Almond Scrub

Ingredients Needed:

- 1/2 cup almond oil
- 1/4 cup ground almonds
- 1/4 cup cornmeal

Directions:

1. Put all the ingredients in a bowl and mix together
2. Apply the scrub to your damp skin in the shower putting more over the particularly dry areas
3. Allow the scrub to soak into your skin for at least 5 minutes
4. Shower yourself clean
5. Pat yourself dry moisturize to keep oils locked into your skin

Refreshing Body Scrubs

We all need a little pick me up now and again and there's no better way than with an invigorating scrub that you have made yourself. Try some of these refreshing recipes, you will love them.

Beautiful Banana Body Scrub

Ingredients Needed:

- 1 ripe banana (when it is starting to turn brown)
- 3 tablespoons brown sugar
- 1 drop rosewood essential oil

Directions:

1. Peel and mash the banana into a bowl
2. Put all the other ingredients in the bowl and mix together
3. Apply the scrub to your damp skin just after you have taken a shower
4. Leave it to work its magic for 5 minutes
5. Shower yourself clean
6. Dry yourself and enjoy how your skin feels

Rejuvenating Citrus Body Scrub

Ingredients Needed:

- 1 cup brown sugar
- 1/2 cup olive oil
- 2 tablespoons lemon essential oil
- 2 tablespoons orange essential oil

Directions:

1. Put all the ingredients in a bowl and mix together.
2. Apply the scrub to your damp skin just after you have taken a shower
3. Allow the scrub to soak into your skin for 5 minutes
4. Shower yourself clean
5. Dry yourself, relax and enjoy how nice your skin feels

Pina Colada Body Scrub

Ingredients Needed:

- 1 cup brown sugar
- 1/2 pineapple (blended)
- 1/2 cup fresh coconut (crushed)
- 4 teaspoons Jojoba oil

Directions:

1. Put all the ingredients in a bowl and mix together.
2. Apply the scrub to your damp skin just after you have taken a shower
3. Allow the scrub to soak into your skin for 5 minutes
4. Shower yourself clean
5. Dry yourself, relax and enjoy how nice your skin feels

Zingy Lime Body Scrub

Ingredients Needed:

- 1 cup sea salt
- 1 lime
- 1/4 cup olive oil

Directions:

1. Cut the lime in half and squeeze the juice out of it
2. Scoop the flesh out and put it in a bowl
3. Add the lime juice, sea salt and olive oil
4. Mix into a paste (add a drop more olive oil if needed)
5. Apply the scrub to your damp skin in the shower
6. Allow the scrub to soak into your skin for 5 minutes
7. Shower yourself clean
8. Dry yourself, relax and enjoy how fresh your skin feels

Penetrating Pomegranate Body Scrub

Ingredients Needed:

- 1 1/2 cups brown sugar
- 1/2 cup groundnut oil
- 1 pomegranate
- 3 drops peppermint essential oil

Directions:

1. Pour the sugar into a bowl and add the pomegranate flesh
2. Add the groundnut and peppermint oils
3. Mix together into a spreadable scrub
4. Apply the scrub to your damp skin in the shower
5. Allow the scrub to soak into your skin for at least 5 minutes
6. Shower yourself clean
7. Dry yourself and enjoy how gorgeous your skin feels

Lazy Ginger Body Scrub

Ingredients Needed:

- 1 tablespoon fresh crushed ginger
- 3/4 cup brown sugar
- 1/4 cup coarse sea salt
- 1/2 cup coconut oil
- 3 drops lime essential oil

Directions:

1. Heat the ginger and the coconut oil in a small pan for 5 minutes on low heat
2. Put the sea salt and brown sugar in a bowl
3. Add the warmed ginger and coconut oil and the drop of lime essential oil
4. Mix into a spreadable scrub
5. Apply the scrub to your damp skin in the shower
6. Allow the scrub to soak into your skin for 5 minutes
7. Shower yourself clean
8. Dry yourself and enjoy how luscious your skin feels

Pure Indulgent Body Scrubs

Why pay tens or hundreds of dollars for a spa treatment when you can create it yourself for pennies? It need not be a special occasion either, treat yourself to an indulgent treatment at least once a week.

ChocoStrawberry Body Scrub

Ingredients Needed:

- 6 tablespoons cocoa powder
- 3 tablespoons brown sugar
- 2 tablespoons coconut oil
- 3 fresh strawberries (crushed)

Directions:

1. Put all the ingredients in a bowl and mix together.
2. Apply the scrub to your damp skin just after you have taken a shower
3. Allow the scrub to soak into your skin for 5 minutes
4. Shower yourself clean
5. Dry yourself, relax and enjoy how polished your skin feels

Sugar & Spice & Everything Nice Body Scrub

Ingredients Needed:

- 1 1/2 cups brown sugar
- 1/2 cup groundnut oil
- 2 teaspoons grated nutmeg
- 2 teaspoons ground cinnamon
- 2 teaspoons ground ginger

Directions:

1. Combine all the ingredients in a bowl and mix together into a spreadable scrub
2. Apply the scrub to your damp skin in the shower
3. Allow the scrub to soak into your skin for 5 minutes
4. Shower yourself clean
5. Dry yourself and enjoy how nice your skin feels

Dead Sea Salt Healthy Scrub

Ingredients Needed:

- 1 cup dead sea salt
- 1/2 cup olive oil
- 4 drops frankincense essential oil

Directions:

1. Put all the ingredients in a bowl and mix together
2. Apply the scrub to your damp skin in the shower
3. Allow the scrub to soak into your skin for 5 minutes
4. Shower yourself clean
5. Pat yourself dry and enjoy your radiant skin

Apple Pie & Custard Body Scrub

Ingredients Needed:

- 1 fresh apple (blend into rough puree)
- 1 cup brown sugar
- 1/2 cup olive oil
- 1/4 cup whole milk
- 2 drops cinnamon essential oil (or 1/2 tsp grated)
- 1/2 tsp grated nutmeg

Directions:

1. Put all the ingredients in a bowl and mix well
2. Apply the scrub to your damp skin in the shower
3. Allow the scrub to soak into your skin for 5 minutes
4. Shower yourself clean
5. Pat yourself dry and enjoy your sweet smelling skin

Deep Vanilla Body Scrub

Ingredients Needed:

- 1/2 cup oats
- 1/2 cup brown sugar
- 1/4 cup olive oil
- 1/4 cup coconut oil
- 1/4 cup hot water
- 3 tablespoons vanilla extract
- 1/2 teaspoon cinnamon

Directions:

1. Put the oatmeal in a bowl and pour the hot water over it
2. When the oats have softened after about 7 minutes add the remaining ingredients
3. Mix together until you get a spreadable paste like consistency
4. Add more sugar if it is a little too runny
5. Apply to your skin when taking a shower
6. Allow the scrub to soak into your skin for 5 minutes
7. Shower yourself clean
8. Pat yourself dry and enjoy your beautiful vanilla scented skin

Fresh Fruit Frenzy Body Scrub

Ingredients Needed:

- 1 cup rolled oats
- 1 medium size banana
- 1 medium size apple
- 1 medium size orange
- 1/4 cup almond oil

Directions:

1. In a bowl, mash the banana with a fork
2. Pulse the apple and orange together in a blender into a paste
3. Add it to the bowl with the banana
4. Add the almond oil and mix together well
5. Apply the scrub to your damp skin in the shower
6. Allow the scrub to soak into your skin for 5 minutes
7. Shower yourself clean
8. Pat yourself dry and enjoy your fruity fresh skin

Coconut, Strawberry & Lemon Body Scrub

Ingredients Needed:

- 1/2 cup brown sugar
- 1/2 cup coconut oil
- 1/4 cup sea salt
- Handful of fresh strawberries
- 4 drops lemon essential oil

Directions:

1. Put the strawberries in a bowl and mash them up with a fork
2. Add all of the other ingredients and mix well into a spreadable paste
3. Add a bit more sea salt if it is too runny or add a little more coconut oil if the consistency is too stiff
4. Apply the scrub to your damp skin when you are in the shower
5. Allow the scrub to soak into your skin for 5 minutes
6. Shower yourself clean
7. Pat yourself dry and enjoy your sweet smelling, beautifully nourished skin

Night Time Body Scrubs

After a stressful day, it is good to be able to get a nice shower or bath and take some much needed rest and relaxation. These night time bath scrubs will get you off to a good start.

Relaxing Lavender & Chamomile Body Scrub

Ingredients Needed:

- 1 cup Epsom salts
- 1/2 cup Coconut Oil
- 4 drops Chamomile essential oil
- 3 drops Lavender essential oil

Directions:

1. Put all the ingredients in a bowl and mix together.
2. Apply the scrub to your damp skin just after you have taken a shower
3. Leave it to work its magic for 5-7 minutes
4. Shower yourself clean
5. Dry yourself and enjoy your beautiful skin

Green Tea & Rosewood Body Scrub

Ingredients Needed:

- 1 cup sea salt
- 1/2 cup Jojoba oil
- 3 organic green tea, teabags
- 4 drops rosewood essential oil

Directions:

1. Snip the green tea teabags open with a pair of scissors and remove the tea
2. Add it to a bowl with all the remaining ingredients and mix together
3. Apply the scrub to your damp skin in the shower
4. Allow the scrub to soak into your skin for 5 minutes
5. Shower yourself clean
6. Pat yourself dry and relax, you deserve it!

Chilling Coconut Body Scrub

Ingredients Needed:

- 1/2 cup coconut oil
- 1/4 cup olive oil
- 3/4 cup natural sea salt
- 1/4 cup brown sugar
- 1/4 cup crushed fresh lavender
- 3 drops lavender essential oil

Directions:

1. Put all the ingredients in a bowl and mix together into a spreadable scrub
2. Apply the scrub to your damp skin in the shower
3. Allow the scrub to soak into your skin for 5 minutes
4. Shower yourself clean
5. Pat yourself dry and chill!

Stress Free Rose Body Scrub

Ingredients Needed:

- 1 cup dead sea salt
- 1/2 cup almond oil
- 1 tablespoon crushed rose petals
- 8 drops rose essential oil

Directions:

1. Put all the ingredients in a bowl and mix together
2. Apply the scrub to your damp skin in the shower
3. Allow the scrub to soak into your skin for 5 minutes
4. Shower yourself clean
5. Pat yourself dry, relax and have a relaxing evening

Cooling Peppermint Sugar Scrub

Ingredients Needed:

- 1 cup ground coffee
- 1/2 cup sea salt
- 6-8 tablespoons olive oil
- 6 drops peppermint essential oil

Directions:

1. Put all the ingredients in a bowl and mix together
2. Apply the scrub to your damp skin in the shower
3. Allow the scrub to soak into your skin for 5 minutes
4. Shower yourself clean
5. Dry yourself, relax and enjoy how nice your skin feels

Calming Rosemary Body Scrub

Ingredients Needed:

- 1 cup dead sea salts
- 3/4 cup coconut oil
- 2 tablespoons fresh rosemary
- 2 drops peppermint essential oil

Directions:

1. Put all the ingredients in a bowl and mix together
2. Apply the scrub to your damp skin in the shower
3. Allow the scrub to soak into your skin for 5 minutes
4. Shower yourself clean
5. Dry yourself, get dressed and relax - you deserve it!

Relaxing Rose Body Scrub

Ingredients Needed:

- 1 1/2 cups brown sugar
- 1 cup coconut oil
- 1 tablespoon Jojoba oil
- Handful of rose petals

Directions:

1. Put all the ingredients in a bowl and mix well
2. Apply the scrub to your damp skin in the shower
3. Allow the scrub to soak into your skin for 5 minutes
4. Shower yourself clean
5. Pat yourself dry and enjoy your rosy skin

Homemade Face Masks

Stop buying expensive store bought face masks or paying for ridiculously priced treatments. Make your own at home with these lovely and easy to prepare recipes.

Honey & Lemon Face Reviver

Ingredients Needed:

- 4 tablespoons brown sugar
- 2 tablespoons honey
- 1 tablespoon olive oil
- 1 teaspoon lemon juice
- 1 tablespoon fresh chopped parsley

Directions:

1. Bash the parsley in a pestle and mortar to release the oils
2. Add to a bowl with all the remaining ingredients and mix together
3. Wash your face
4. Apply the mask to your face and leave it on for 5-7 minutes
5. Wash it off your face
6. Pat your face dry and just see how clean and revitalized your skin feels

Rosemary & Lavender Face Smoother

Ingredients Needed:

- 4 tablespoons fine brown sugar
- 2-3 tablespoons coconut oil
- 2 tablespoons fresh lavender
- 2 tablespoon fresh rosemary

Directions:

1. Put all the ingredients in a bowl and mix together
2. Wash your face
3. Apply the scrub, gently rubbing into the skin in circular motions working from the bottom of your face to the top
4. Allow the scrub to work its magic on your face for 5 minutes
5. Wash the scrub off your face
6. Pat your face dry, look in the mirror and smile at the look and feel of your radiant skin

Natural Yogurt Face Toning Mask

Ingredients Needed:

- 1 tablespoon brown sugar
- 1/4 teaspoon honey
- 1 tablespoon natural yogurt

Directions:

1. Put all the ingredients in a bowl and mix together
2. Wash your face
3. Apply face mask and allow to penetrate your skin for 5 minutes
4. Wash the scrub off
5. Pat yourself face dry and moisturize with your favorite cream

Coffee Complexion Restorer

Ingredients Needed:

- 4 tablespoons ground coffee
- 4 tablespoons cocoa powder
- 8 tablespoons coconut oil
- 1 teaspoon honey

Directions:

1. Put all the ingredients in a bowl and mix together
2. Apply the scrub to your face and massage all over
3. Leave and allow the scrub to soak into your face for 5 minutes
4. Wash your face with warm water
5. Pat dry and enjoy your refreshed skin

Easy Egg Face Mask

Ingredients Needed:

- Whites of 2 large eggs
- 2 tablespoons of plain yogurt

Directions:

1. Mix the egg whites and yogurt in a bowl to form a smooth paste
2. Wash your face
3. Apply the face mask and let it penetrate for 5 minutes
4. Wash it off with warm water
5. Pat dry and enjoy your tighter toned face

Strawberry Shiner Face Mask

Ingredients Needed:

- 1 teaspoon lemon juice
- 1 egg white
- 1/2 teaspoon honey
- 1/2 cup fresh strawberries

Directions:

1. Put all the ingredients in a bowl and mix together
2. Wash your face
3. Apply the mask to your face and allow to penetrate into your pores for 5 minutes
4. Wash the mask off with warm water
5. Rinse your face with cold water
6. Enjoy your lovely shinier smooth complexion

Oatmeal & Baking Soda Face Mask

Ingredients Needed:

- 1 tablespoon oatmeal
- 1 tablespoon baking soda
- 2 tablespoons warm water

Directions:

1. Pour the oatmeal into a bowl and add the warm water
2. Allow the oatmeal to soften a bit and add the baking soda
3. Mix together to form a paste
4. Wash your face
5. Put the mask on your face and allow to penetrate your skin for 5 minutes
6. Wash off with warm water
7. Feel your super soft face

Homemade Lip Balms

Chapped, cracked or rough lips will be a thing of the past with these wonderful lip balm recipes. Protect and treat your lips the way they should be treated, with love, care and attention.

Simple Shea Lip Balm

Ingredients Needed:

- 4g beeswax
- 5g shea butter
- 3g cocoa butter
- 4g olive oil
- 4g avocado oil
- 3 drops vitamin E oil
- 4 drops of your favorite essential oil

Directions:

1. Pour all the ingredients (except the essential oil) into a small pan
2. Allow the ingredients to fuse together until melted (low heat)
3. Add your favorite essential oils once the mixture has melted and cooled a bit
4. Pour into a small air tight jar or into lip balm tubes if you have any
5. Enjoy your luscious lip balm and gorgeous soft lips

Coconut Softening Lip Moisturizer

Ingredients Needed:

- 1 tablespoon grated beeswax
- 1 tablespoon coconut oil
- 1/2 tablespoon honey
- 2 vitamin E capsules

Directions:

1. In a small bowl, melt the beeswax in the microwave in 5 second bursts until fully melted
2. Remove from the heat and add the coconut oil and honey
3. Add the inside of the vitamin E capsules
4. Pour into a small air tight jar or into lip balm tubes if you have any
5. Allow to cool
6. Enjoy your sweet coconut lip balm

Easy Anti Chapping Mint Balm

Ingredients Needed:

- 1 tablespoon Vaseline
- 3 drops peppermint essential oil

Directions:

1. Mix the Vaseline and peppermint oil together
2. Pour into a small air tight jar, lip balm tin or lip balm tubes if you have any
3. Allow to infuse for an hour
4. Enjoy your luscious lip balm and gorgeous soft lips

Luxurious Lavender Lip Balm

Ingredients Needed:

- 4 tablespoons Jojoba oil
- 1 tablespoon grated beeswax
- 1 teaspoon honey
- 2 vitamin E capsules
- 7 drops lavender essential oil

Directions:

1. Pour the Jojoba oil, beeswax and honey into a small pan and allow to blend on low heat
2. Allow the ingredients to fuse together until all the beeswax has melted (low heat)
3. Add the content of the vitamin E capsules
4. Remove from heat, allow to cool for 5 minutes and add the lavender essential oil
5. Pour into a small air tight jar or tins and allow to harden for a few hours
6. Enjoy your luscious lip balm and gorgeous soft lips

Healing Geranium Lip Balm

Ingredients Needed:

- 4g beeswax
- 5g shea butter
- 6g avocado oil
- 3 drops vitamin E oil
- 4 drops geranium essential oil

Directions:

1. Pour the beeswax, shea butter and avocado oil into a pan
2. Allow the ingredients to fuse together until you can see the beeswax has melted
3. Add the vitamin E oil and geranium essential oil
4. Mix together well
5. Pour into a small air tight jar or tin
6. Enjoy your healing lip balm

Mellow Mango Lip Balm

Ingredients Needed:

- 1/4 oz cocoa butter
- 1/4 oz shea butter
- 1/4 oz mango butter
- 2 tablespoons beeswax
- 5ml mango flavored oil

Directions:

1. Pour all the ingredients into a small bowl and melt in microwave in 10 second intervals
2. Once completely melted, pour into small air tight jars or tins.
3. Allow to set for a minimum of 4 hours
4. Enjoy your mellow mango lips

Homemade Body Washes

Whatever you put on your body seeps into your system so only use the best natural ingredients, you deserve it after all. These homemade body wash recipes will have you wondering how you managed without them for so long.

Natural Honey Body Wash

Ingredients Needed:

- 2/3 cup natural liquid soap
- 1/4 cup raw honey
- 2 teaspoons sweet almond oil
- 1 teaspoon vitamin E oil
- 6 drops chamomile essential oil

Directions:

1. Put all the ingredients in a bottle (with a lid) and mix together
2. Shake it up again just before you use it
3. Get in the shower or bath and wash your skin with this luscious honey wash
4. Rinse off and pat yourself dry
5. Enjoy the wonderful benefits of natural honey on your skin

Your Favorite Soap Body Wash

Ingredients Needed:

- 6 cups natural spring or mineral water
- 3 bars natural soap (grated) or your favorite soap (grated)

Directions:

1. Put all the ingredients in a pan and stir on low to medium heat until all the soap has dissolved
2. Transfer the liquid to a glass jar and allow it to cool
3. Put it in a plastic body wash bottle, place it by the shower and use it at your leisure

Coconut Milk Body Wash

Ingredients Needed:

- 1/2 cup coconut oil liquid soap (grated finely)
- 1/3 cup coconut milk
- 2 drops sweet almond oil
- 8 drops chamomile essential oil

Directions:

1. Put all the ingredients in a plastic body wash bottle and shake to combine the ingredients
2. Place it by the shower and use it at your leisure
3. You will have to shake it up a bit when you want to use it again
4. Enjoy your coconut body wash

Herb Infusion Body Wash

Ingredients Needed:

- 1/2 cup liquid soap
- 10 drops rosemary essential oil
- 8 drops lavender essential oil
- 6 drops chamomile essential oil
- 4 drops peppermint essential oil

Directions:

1. Pour all ingredients into a plastic body wash bottle and stir vigorously
2. Place it by the shower and use it at your leisure
3. Shake before each use

Lush Lavender Body Wash

Ingredients Needed:

- 3 cups natural spring or mineral water
- 1/4 cup Aloe Vera gel
- 1/4 cup olive oil
- 1/4 cup coconut oil
- 1 tablespoon shea butter
- 1 cup guar gum
- 1 cup Dr Bronner's Castile soap
- 4 drops lavender essential oil

Directions:

1. Put all the ingredients in a blender (except the castile soap)
2. Blend on high for 60 seconds
3. Stir in castile soap and mix well
4. Pour into a plastic body wash bottle, place it by the shower and use it at your leisure

Tea Tree Body Wash

Ingredients Needed:

- 1/4 cup Dr Bronner's Castile soap
- 3/4 cup water
- 6 drops Tea Tree essential oil
- 2 tablespoons glycerin
- 1 bar natural soap (grated) or your favorite moisturizing soap (grated)

Directions:

1. Melt and pour all ingredients into a plastic body wash bottle and shake vigorously,
2. Place it by the shower and use it at your leisure

Conclusion

Well, I have given you 52 of my favorite natural homemade recipes and have also given you an insight into the dangers in continuing to use some of those store bought products.

You now know how easy they are to put together so get started straight away and try some of them out. The more you make and use them, the more you will grow to love them just like me.

If you are treating a particular skin condition, concentrate on recipes that are relevant to that. Make your own combinations too by studying further the health benefits of the salts, sugars and oils I use and also the essential oils which are super important too.

Thank you for reading and I hope you have enjoyed this book as much as I have enjoyed putting it together for you.

Lorraine xx

Don't forget to take a look at my other books in this series, all available on Amazon

- **Homemade Lotions:** 41 All Natural, Simple & Easy To Make Body Lotions, Body Butters & Lotion Bars

- **How To Make Bath Bombs:** *Bath Salts & Bubble Baths: 53 All Natural & Organic Recipes*

- **Homemade Beauty Products:** Over 50 All Natural Recipes For Face Masks, Facial Cleansers & Face Creams: Natural Organic Recipes For Youthful Skin

- **Homemade Foot Spa:** 48 All Natural Foot Scrubs, Foot Soaks, Foot Creams & Heel Balm Recipes

27811764R00046

Made in the USA
Middletown, DE
22 December 2015